MANAGING HYPERSENSITIVITY IN CHILDREN AND ADULTS

Exercises and practical advice to help
hypersensitive people understand their emotions
and live happily without effort.

———————

Christelle Chartier

Summary

Preface

Hello, dear reader! If you have this book in your hands, it's probably because you have questions about hypersensitivity. Maybe you recognize yourself in these descriptions of people who feel everything a little too intensely, or maybe you're trying to understand a loved one who lives with this characteristic. Anyway, welcome! You are in the right place.

Why this book?

Imagine yourself in a room full of people, where every sound, every light, every emotion seems amplified. For some, it's just a normal situation, but for you, it's a sensory and emotional roller coaster. Hypersensitivity is a bit like that: a mixture of intensity and heightened perception that can be both wonderful and exhausting. We wrote this book to help you navigate this world with a little more clarity and a lot more kindness towards yourself.

What will we discover together?

We will explore what hypersensitivity is in all its facets. You will discover touching anecdotes and concrete examples that will perhaps make you smile or feel less alone. We will talk about the daily challenges that hypersensitive people encounter and, above all, strategies to overcome them. No complicated jargon here, just practical advice and clear explanations so you can really understand and take action.

Real stories and practical advice

This book is full of stories of people who have learned to live with their hypersensitivity, sometimes even to take advantage of it. Their experiences show that, despite obstacles, it is possible to flourish. You will also find practical advice, relaxation techniques, tips for organizing your daily life and methods for better managing your emotions.

A casual but serious tone

We wanted this book to be like a conversation with a friend – accessible, warm, and above all, useful. Hypersensitivity can be a challenge, but with the right information and a little humor, it can also become a real strength. Our goal is to provide you with concrete tools so that you can transform your sensitivity into an asset.

Forward, together!

So, are you ready for this adventure? Whether you are hypersensitive yourself or looking to help a loved one, this book is for you. Together, let's discover how to transform the challenges of hypersensitivity into a positive force in your life.

Welcome to this exploration. Take a deep breath, relax, and dive into this guide. You are about to discover a world where hypersensitivity is no longer an obstacle, but a facet of what makes you unique and incredible.

Good reading !

Chapter 1

Understanding Hypersensitivity

The question that arises is what hypersensitivity actually represents. It is a unique and exquisite presence of hyperconsciousness to the world, to others and even to the invisible elements of our environment. Hypersensitivity involves a high ability to detect cognitive, intuitive, and sensory information; it describes individuals who react much more intensely than others to stimuli in their environment eliciting vivid and distinctly distinct emotional responses based on atypical brain functionality and heightened intuitive abilities.

Hypersensitivity is not a disease; it is a quality that is revealed through increased sensitivity to one's environment. "Hyper" in hypersensitivity means "beyond the ordinary," and when we say "sensitive," we mean the ability to sense or perceive accurately. This implies that we feel emotions much more intensely than others and that we cannot protect ourselves from the feelings of those around us, whether people near or far. Highly sensitive individuals are extremely delicate and refined, often thriving in creative atmospheres. There are different forms of hypersensitivity:

Hypersensitivity is not just higher than normal sensitivity: it applies to both sensory and emotional levels. Hyperemotionality defines all aspects of life, but particularly romantic relationships, where the singularity of both partners can be fully expressed. It is often considered an inconvenience in daily life; something that can lead to pain. However, turning your hypersensitivity into strength is well within your reach. A hypersensitive person will show an exaggerated response to sensory stimuli: all five senses might be involved in stimuli that others don't even notice. Hyperemotional people tend to have increased empathy, but also experience more intense and diverse emotions on a daily basis than most people. Hyperemotionality may also involve specific cognitive traits, such as an increased inclination toward contemplation and cognitive or introspective analysis, characteristics that are often dominant in these individuals. This acuity of perception can, particularly in relationships, lead to distress, as these individuals tend to grasp the subtleties of interaction situations on both rational and emotional levels. In other words, they sometimes understand the difficulty in managing their emotions even when they perceive the subtle elements that compose them.

Four types of hypersensitivity reactions are known: type i, type ii, type iii and type iv.

The main types of hypersensitivity reactions are classified into four broad categories. In the first type, called immediate hypersensitivity (type I) or allergy, the damage is caused by TH2 cells, IgE antibodies, mast cells and other leukocytes. Mast cells release mediators that have vasoactive properties acting on blood vessels and smooth muscles, as well as cytokines that promote and activate inflammatory cells at the site of injury. The second category is antibody-mediated disorders (type II hypersensitivity), in which secreted IgG and IgM antibodies bind to antigens present on tissues or cell surfaces. Antibodies act in different ways: they can cause cell destruction by phagocytosis or lysis induced by inflammation signals; interfere with cellular functions even if no structural damage occurs (as in autoimmunity); lead to disease without direct effect on cells or tissues.

Type I hypersensitivity is also known as immediate hypersensitivity and generally follows a specific sequence of events in cellular responses. This involves the activation of TH2 cells leading to the production of IgE antibodies. Allergens can be introduced into the body by inhalation, ingestion or injection.

Factors that play a role in strong TH2 responses to allergens include the route, dose, and chronicity of exposure as well as host genetics. Whether allergenic substances have unique properties at the structural or chemical level that allow them to induce TH2 responses remains unclear, but immediate hypersensitivity serves as an example of a TH2-mediated reaction where induced TH2 cells produce cytokines such as IL-4, IL-5 and IL-13 which cause most of the reactions responsible for this type of hypersensitivity. Among these cytokines, IL-4 acts on allergen-specific B cells by promoting the switch to the IgE heavy chain class, resulting in the production and secretion of IgE immunoglobulins.

Allergic reactions that occur shortly after exposure to an allergen are called immediate or type I hypersensitivity. Let's look at penicillin allergy, which is a common manifestation of this type of hypersensitivity. Other topics related to hypersensitivity include Type II (cytotoxic) hypersensitivity exemplified by pemphigus vulgaris, Type III hypersensitivity (immune complexes), and Type IV (or delayed) exemplified by lichen planus or HS type IV against latex with lymphoblastic. Transform test (TTL). We will also discuss hypersensitivity states of innate immunity during this exploration. Symptoms and manifestations are key elements when examining cases of hypersensitivity: they must always be taken into account when making a diagnosis!

Hypersensitivity can take many forms. We separate hyperesthesia (defining increased sensitivity of the senses – hearing, sight, smell, touch, etc.) from emotional hypersensitivity which will be discussed in more detail here. Sensory and emotional hypersensitivity: two distinct aspects of the same phenomenon.

Drug hypersensitivity is an immune response. Symptoms vary in severity and may take the form of rash, anaphylaxis, or serum sickness. The diagnosis is generally clinical; although skin testing is sometimes helpful. Treatment involves stopping the medication; Supportive treatment (e.g. antihistamines) should also be taken and in some cases desensitization may be used.

Hypersensitivity is not easy to live with; but recognizing the strength that comes from it can make a big difference. Converting this sensitivity into personal strength will lead you to more open doors in your life.

Causes and triggers of hypersensitivity reactions.

Hypersensitivity acts as an amplifier of all experiences, leading to increased reactivity to any form of stimuli, whether they originate from within (such as thoughts or physical conditions like stomach upset, digestion or menstruation) or the external environment.

The slightly stimulating thus proves very stimulating for people with a high level of sensitivity. It goes without saying that what can create distress for the majority becomes completely traumatic for an individual with hypersensitivity traits.

Hypersensitivity occurs when the immune response does not match the level of threat posed by the intruder, which can include a range of substances such as bacteria, viruses, toxins, endotoxins or allergens. The reaction takes place in three stages: first the sensitization phase (initial exposure to the antigen), then a latency period where the immunological processes of the reaction take place; and finally, the actual tissue damage during the second contact (which acts as a trigger with the antigen) takes place at another stage.

An immediate hypersensitivity reaction (type I) may occur in response to a systemic disorder or a local reaction. The type and extent of the reaction is often dictated by the route of exposure to the antigen. Systemic exposure to protein antigens such as those found in bee venom or drugs such as penicillin can lead to what is known as systemic anaphylaxis. This usually manifests within minutes of exposure in a sensitized person with symptoms of pruritus, urticaria and erythematous skin changes, all warning signs of imminent bronchoconstriction which will quickly manifest as dyspnea with wheezing. audible due to damage to the airways by bronchospasm and laryngeal obstruction. Hypersecretion and mucous plugs aggravate problems at the bronchiolar level, which adds distal resistance to other areas of higher resistance located up to the vocal cords.

Hypersensitivity – the scourge of everyday life. The constant assault on our senses can turn even the simplest tasks into herculean feats. Think about nails on a chalkboard all day and every day. Does this seem too hard? Imagine a bright light that seems to pierce your retinas with every glance. These are just small examples of how hypersensitivity can completely derail an otherwise normal day. Whether it's avoiding certain fabrics because they feel like sandpaper against your skin or avoiding crowded places because of overwhelming noise levels, every decision is dictated by this condition. And yet, despite its pervasive impact, hypersensitivity is often misunderstood or worse, completely ignored by those who do not experience it themselves. The next time someone jumps at the sound of a door opening or grimaces when you accidentally brush past them in a crowded space, remember this: To them, these everyday events are anything but insignificant.

Living with hypersensitivity on a daily basis is no walk in the park. Often we find ourselves at odds with our reactions, unsure why we act the way we do, or feeling guilty for being passive in uncontrollable situations. We can feel attacked by noise, by people, or conversely be bored by lack of external stimulation. Essentially, being hypersensitive involves accepting who you are; it calls for self-awareness and self-acceptance. So love yourself when you deserve it, but also don't hesitate to challenge yourself when needed. It's all part of the journey to understanding and accepting your hypersensitive self.

Finding balance with your heightened sensitivity can be difficult on a daily basis, but it is entirely possible to thrive with this overflow of emotions. In order not to let yourself be swallowed up by this hyper sensitivity, simple psychotherapeutic techniques exist, they can help protect yourself, especially during social interactions. Finding the key within yourself: it's the secret to feeling good about yourself and, consequently, being good to others.

Indeed, hypersensitivity (which includes hyperemotionality) can be extremely intense for those who experience it daily. It's always enriching to have different perspectives on the subject. It can help us understand and, more importantly, support our child. They too are forced to navigate through their emotions which push them to improvise and grow day by day.

Hypersensitivity in children and adults differs in this way: the increasingly frequent phenomena are those of hypersensitive children and adults whose level of sensitivity is much higher than that of the average so-called sensitive people, but who at the same time also tends to be more or less expressed, controlled or repressed.

There are variations in sensitivity among children. For those who struggle to deal with overwhelming emotions on their own, how can a parent identify such a child? What factors contribute to hypersensitivity? In what ways can parents help their hypersensitive child?

A child fails to control his or her emotions and is therefore called hypersensitive because emotions take over. Its sensory channels are developed above the ordinary level; he perceives what he experiences with a higher intensity than others. "A hypersensitive child is a child who has sensors open to the world. In addition to his own emotions, he perceives those of those around him and the energies of the places where he evolves.

Category	Description	Examples
Features		
Emotional sensitivity	Intense emotional reactions to external and internal stimuli	Crying easily while watching movies, feeling overwhelmed with emotion in social situations
Increased empathy	Ability to deeply feel the emotions of others	Feeling a friend's sadness as if it were your own, being strongly affected by conflicts
Sensory sensitivity	Increased reactions to sensory stimuli such as light, sound and textures	Being disturbed by bright lights, loud noises, or rough fabrics
Deep reflection	Tendency to think intensely about experiences and emotions	Analyze social interactions at length, rehash conversations
Need for solitude	Need for alone time to recharge and recover	Retreat to a quiet room after intense social interactions

Chapter 2

Identifying Hypersensitivity

Revealing the signs and symptoms of hypersensitivity is a step towards better understanding. Hypersensitivity: telltale signs and symptoms.

This feeling of being able to "feel" others and connect with them on a deeper level is what defines hypersensitivity. The highly sensitive person picks up these signals by carefully observing details and any changes in the other person's mood or physical expression, which can serve as clear indicators of underlying emotion. Interestingly, these same elements can also suggest high intellectual potential.

High sensitivity alludes to alternative world perception, distinct modes of interaction, and divergent cognitive processes. As a result, responses may appear exaggerated or disproportionate to what is considered normal. This increased sensitivity affects all spheres of life (relational, emotional, sensory) and manifests itself through the child's actions and emotions that arise from their environment. Hypersensitivity may be genetic with variable changes over time; this implies that it continually evolves and indirectly impacts all aspects of the child's development.

There's nothing more infuriating than hypersensitivity, especially when it surprises you and you don't understand why your reactions are so much fiercer than others. Such a condition can elicit fear in an individual, leading them to avoid new experiences out of apprehension of their reaction, or to withdraw from social scenarios to avoid potential humiliation.

Two types of hypersensitivity reactions: immediate and delayed.

Two types of hypersensitivity are distinguished depending on time: hypersensitivity can occur immediately or later. Immediate hypersensitivity will elicit an emotional or behavioral response at that moment. Delayed hypersensitivity frequently associated with previous events or trauma will manifest its response later upon exposure to reactivating stimuli.

Allergic disorders (such as atopic disorders) and other hypersensitivity diseases are immune reactions. They occur when the body overreacts or inappropriately to foreign antigens.

Another form of inappropriate immune response occurs when the immune system acts against the body's own components (autoimmune disorders).

Children are no exception and present with obvious signs and symptoms. Overall, highly sensitive individuals need more time than others to adapt to change; it is important that those around them understand them so that the changes can be experienced as calmly as possible and that they can be supported during this long period of adaptation. This includes children who have obvious signs and symptoms, so make sure you know what they are.

The signals are not exclusive to hypersensitivity. They may be in your child's home for other reasons; If you notice several of these signals, plus difficulty managing your emotions, or if you witness a lot of crying or excessive anger every day, do not hesitate to consult a mental health professional or pediatrician to find out more. the situation.

The child's reactions to these elements may be stronger, but also disproportionate to other people around him. However, we must realize that these responses are not due to a desire (whim), but to a known disorder.

Symptoms manifest either dermatologically (notably tingling, hot sensations, itching and redness) or neurologically (headaches, dizziness, fatigue) or cognitive problems such as memory loss, but they occur in various other systems such as the gastrointestinal or cardiovascular systems. Some studies have focused on distinguishing two subgroups of hypersensitive patients based on how they attribute the problem. The first group complains of skin problems related to computer work, with most symptoms localized on the face, transient in nature and showing a positive response on weekends or after working hours. Another subgroup presents symptoms related to electrical devices, hence the name "electrical hypersensitivity," a more recent and less well-defined syndrome. The outlook is rather bleak if attempts at mitigation through remedial measures prove unsuccessful; this generally leads to an escalation of avoidance behaviors resulting in an inability to work sometimes associated with marked social isolation .

Clinical signs and symptoms in adults.

Neurovegetative symptoms are more common in older hypersensitive people, although the majority of them are between 40 and 50 years old. Scandinavian studies report a higher incidence of hypersensitive environments in women than in men, which contrasts with data from a California study that was conducted among the general population, focusing on people self-identified as being electrically hypersensitive individuals. The search for a pathophysiological marker linked to this pathology remains inconclusive. As highlighted by a study looking at cholinesterase activity that showed no reduction, fatigue in people hypersensitive to electricity is still under investigation for any potential association with exposure to fields. electromagnetic. Application of antioxidant treatments (such as vitamin C, E, and selenium) to individuals suspected of being hypersensitive does not result in improvement in symptoms or serum oxidative status. Differences have been observed in some dermatological and histopathological parameters , including the number and distribution of mast cells in the dermis by different investigators with varying results. Melatonin has received little attention despite being the most commonly cited hormone in relation to the health effects of electromagnetic fields. There is therefore little information regarding its study in relation to HE. The European report tells stories of contradictions: sometimes stories of increased melatonin in these hypersensitive patients, showing dermatological and neurasthenic symptoms, while others tell stories of contradictions. Tales where no difference is found between hypersensitive souls and healthy beings.

Common triggers for hypersensitivity reactions: presence of strong odors, air conditioning and cigarette smoke, odors (e.g., perfumes, cleaning products), sudden exposure to bright light.

Hypersensitivity is an extreme response to any type of internal or external stimulation, whether emotional, sensory or physical. Only a few stimuli can be perceived as very intense by sensitive individuals, which others often do not notice. This increased sensitivity manifests itself in various forms.

Hypersensitivity is a phenomenon in which the immune response does not match the level of threat posed by the intruder which may be a bacteria, virus, toxin, endotoxin or allergen. The evolution of the hypersensitivity reaction takes place in three phases: first the sensitization phase (the first contact with the antigen), then comes a latency phase where the immunological mechanisms are established and finally we have a lesion phase during which there is another contact on trigger with the antigen.

Hypersensitivity is more than just exaggerated responses to stimuli; it goes far beyond the emotional and sensory realms, even surpassing physical limits. It has a profound impact on the daily lives of those who encounter it. When we recognize these particular sensitivities, showing empathy and trying to grasp them with understanding, we take small steps towards inclusion in our practices as a society, where the needs of each individual can be recognized without judgment nor prejudices.

Importance of early detection and appropriate control of hypersensitivity cases.

Diagnosis of hypersensitivity involves a detailed assessment that incorporates self-assessment, clinical observation, interviews, history review, and interdisciplinary teamwork. There is no single medical test; However, mental health experts discover hypersensitivity traits from an individual's response to emotions, patterns of social dynamics, and personal or family history. It is important to understand that hypersensitivity is simply considered a personality characteristic rather than a clinical condition. Nonetheless, the repercussions of hypersensitivity can significantly affect a person's well-being, primarily emotional and psychological aspects that might require therapeutic intervention to help individuals better manage their hypersensitive nature.

Learning to identify and change the thoughts and beliefs that fuel control and perfectionism can also be vital for the highly sensitive. By challenging these thought patterns, they are able to adapt a more flexible outlook on life.

Hypersensitivity is not considered a disease in itself, so there is no direct treatment that can be prescribed. However, delving into the realm of emotion management and combatting stress can play a pivotal role in enabling highly sensitive people to lead better lives through their unique emotional sensitivity.

Category	Potential Cause	Description
Genetic		
Family history	Hypersensitivity present in other family members	Having parents, grandparents or siblings with hypersensitive traits
Genetic polymorphisms	Genetic variations that can affect sensory processing	Genes influencing the nervous system and emotional reactions
Neurobiology		
Functioning of the nervous system	Differences in how the brain processes	More reactive nervous system,

	sensory and emotional stimuli	increased response to external stimuli
Hyperactivation of the amygdala	Increased emotional reactivity	More active brain amygdala, amplifying emotional responses and stress
Development and Environment		
Early experiences	Significant childhood experiences	Childhood marked by stressful, traumatic or, on the contrary, very protective events
Family environment	Parenting style and family atmosphere	Growing in a very stressful or hyperprotective environment
Psychology and Personality		
Personality traits	Innate Personality Characteristics	Introspective nature, tendency towards

		deep reflection, increased emotional sensitivity
Traumatic experiences	Stressful or traumatic events experienced	Experiencing trauma (physical or emotional) increasing emotional sensitivity
Culture and Society		
Cultural norms	Societal expectations and values	Growing up in a culture that values emotional expression or repression of emotions
Social support	Level of social support and acceptance	Social environment understanding and supportive or, on the contrary, critical and unempathetic
Health and wellbeing		

Chronic stress level	Prolonged exposure to stress	Living in a state of constant stress, affecting emotional and sensory reactivity
Sleep and diet	Quality of sleep and diet	Poor sleep and unbalanced diet exacerbate emotional and physical reactions

Chapter 3

The Challenges of Hypersensitivity

Hypersensitivity is an art. Accepting it as part of our being while recognizing its existence can lead us to explore unexplored potentials and thus make peace with it. Numerous documentary resources, testimonies and interactions with other hypersensitive people help us in this journey.

Take control of your hypersensitivity: find the signs of hypersensitivity that belong to you. This can manifest as overwhelming emotional responses or a magnet-like absorption of others' emotions, even causing physical weariness due to environmental factors. Being able to recognize these signs will help you better manage your own reactivity.

Living conditions can make life difficult for hypersensitive people, which can manifest as extreme reactivity to sensory, emotional, and social stimuli. Hypersensitivity can manifest in a variety of forms, including increased sensitivity to light or noise or difficulty understanding the emotions of others or being contemplative about personal experiences.

Adaptability Advantage: Highly sensitive individuals are able to adapt quickly due to their ability to absorb a large amount of information with their highly responsive brains, allowing them to process information more deeply. Often intuitive, they can spot problems before they materialize.

The adaptability of highly sensitive people is generally exceptional. When scuba diving, various challenges present themselves; for example, water pressure and limited visibility as well as currents. In these situations, highly sensitive people can use their adaptive skills to quickly understand and respond to the ever-changing underwater environment.

The impact of hypersensitivity on personal relationships can be devastating, as highly sensitive people easily feel overwhelmed by a multitude of sensory, emotional, and environmental stimuli. To deal with this, it is crucial to establish a peaceful and relaxing environment. This may involve seeking out quiet alone time, engaging in calming activities such as meditation or yoga to relax, and setting limits on what depletes your energy reserves by finding ways to keep them at bay for self-preservation.

Hypersensitivity tends to surface in specific scenarios. As a result, the person who struggles with hypersensitivity in interpersonal relationships has difficulty rationalizing their emotions, putting them in context, or searching for the intention behind them. Additionally, decision-making becomes a complex task for these people. Highly sensitive individuals generally possess a keen sense of observation, an attribute that makes them very attentive. This increased level of attention allows them to pick up on stimuli that would otherwise escape the attention of the people around them…except themselves. These same stimuli also have the ability to elicit an extremely intense emotional response within them, further complicating matters.

A high level of sensitivity can greatly hinder healthy social interactions, as individuals may struggle to communicate effectively. It is true that the hypersensitive individual hates conflicts, which usually arise from different negative thoughts and lead to inner confusion and increased anxiety levels. As a result, this person is more likely to internalize the responsibility to avoid actions that might hurt or provoke anger in others, often leading to feeling frustrated (or even resentful) toward them later.

In the area of interpersonal relationships, highly sensitive people demonstrate an innate talent for establishing deep relationships with others. Their keen empathy and sensitivity allows them to accurately feel and grasp the emotions of those around them. They are wise and caring listeners, a trait which in turn fosters authentic and meaningful relationships.

Tactics for controlling hypersensitivity in the workplace.

There are ways to reduce stress by creating a more relaxed and supportive workspace. One such strategy is to take regular breaks during work hours to revitalize yourself, another is to design a calm work environment where everything is in its place and free of any clutter that could increase your stress levels. Communicate openly with your colleagues and superiors so that they understand your situation and provide you with the necessary support.

A few strategies allow you to not only alleviate the discomfort of hypersensitivity, but also to see this increased sensitivity as a strength rather than a weakness. Here are some tips for managing hypersensitivity in the professional sphere:

Managing hypersensitivity at work requires mastering emotional control and isolating oneself from stimuli external to oneself. There are several methods to do this: relaxation techniques, therapy sessions or simply learning to say no when necessary. For a calmer work environment, highly sensitive people may also seek accommodations to reduce disruptive stimuli.

When dealing with hypersensitivity in children, one should consider engaging them in creative and sensory activities that would help them divert their energy and express their emotions in a positive way. It is important that these children are exposed to different artistic forms whether it is painting, drawing, music or dance, as these mediums allow for free self-expression.

Hypersensitivity in children is an often overlooked problem, but it is a real problem that could significantly affect their emotions and daily lives. When triggered by external stimuli—loud noises, bright lights, textures, or even the emotions of others — hypersensitive children react in very strong and profound ways.

A child's hypersensitivity is marked by a heightened awareness of their own emotions as well as those of those around them, often associated with heightened sensory experiences that can be upsetting. Hypersensitivity, which affects 20% of the population, is not a disease: would it be absurd to consider increased empathy towards others as pathological? However, this provokes responses in the child that may seem excessive or unjustified, leading to harmful effects on their relationships, emotions and sensory aspects. So many contributing factors despite its non-pathological nature. An affliction that is not an illness and that causes suffering? In such circumstances, it becomes crucial to be attuned to the child's emotional world in order to enable them to make the most of this heightened sensitivity they possess.

Emotional and behavioral challenges in hypersensitive adults.

Highly sensitive adults are more sensitive to their emotions and those of others, so they feel emotions with greater intensity and are easily overwhelmed by them. The emotional palette is richer and more varied than that of other individuals: this trait is called hyper emotionality, also characteristic of people with high potential (HPI or HPE). This emotional richness is not understood by everyone; it can lead to deep suffering and a feeling of loneliness. It would then be useful to associate yourself with other hypersensitive people who understand what you are going through, so that you do not feel alone.

Demands for balance and self-care: Highly sensitive people typically develop a strong demand for balance and self-care in their daily lives. Because of this heightened emotional sensitivity, they are more likely to experience stress that could easily lead to burnout. However, they are aware of their needs and the importance of being able to find the right ways to recharge their batteries in the way that suits them best. Whether through wellness practices or finding time for their hobbies, they recognize these moments with value and make time without compromise.

Understanding empathy towards others can be defined as an innate quality of highly sensitive adults in that they can understand their emotions and those of others. And the very sensitive people with whom they come into contact are able to place great trust in them without any difficulty; trust comes spontaneously to these people who easily confide in the most sensitive. Highly sensitive individuals have high levels of awareness and are able to read the emotional needs of those around them. They offer support by lending an empathetic ear, which makes many highly sensitive people good caregivers, doctors, therapists, etc.

Category	Challenges	Description	Potential Consequences
Emotions			
Intense emotional reactions	Dealing with strong and sudden emotions	Feeling emotions like joy, sadness, anger or fear very intensely	Emotional exhaustion, difficulty controlling reactions, anxiety and depression
Increased empathy	Absorbing the emotions of others	Deeply feeling the emotions of loved ones, friends or even strangers	Emotional overwork, difficulty establishing personal boundaries
Sensitivity to criticism	React strongly to negative comments	Feeling hurt by criticism, even constructive criticism	Lower self-esteem, avoidance of constructive feedback
Physical sensations			
Sensory sensitivity	Dealing with increased	Being easily disturbed by loud noises, bright lights,	Increased stress and anxiety, avoidance of

	sensory stimuli	strong smells or unpleasant textures	stimulating environments
Intense physical reactions	Reacting strongly to pain, hunger or fatigue	Exacerbated feeling of physical sensations	Difficulty concentrating, increased fatigue, irritability

Social

Exhausting social interactions	Feeling quickly exhausted by social interactions	Needing to retreat from social interactions to recharge	Social isolation, difficulty maintaining social relationships
Conflict sensitivity	Avoiding or being very affected by conflicts	Feeling intense emotional distress during arguments or conflicts	Avoidance of confrontations, accumulation of resentment

Professional

Managing stress at work	React strongly to stress and job expectations	Feeling overwhelmed by deadlines, criticism, or stressful work environments	Burn-out, decline in performance, difficulty maintaining a job

Concentration and productivity	Maintaining concentration in distracting work environments	Being easily distracted by environmental stimuli	Reduced productivity, frequent errors, frustration
Emotional and psychological			
Anxiety and depression	Increased risk of anxiety and depressive disorders	Feeling constant worry and depressive episodes	Difficulty functioning in daily life, need for medical or therapeutic treatment
Excessive self-criticism	Being very critical of yourself	Blaming yourself disproportionately for minor mistakes	Lower self-esteem, paralyzing perfectionism
Well-being and Health			
Sleep quality	Difficulty getting restful sleep	Having trouble falling asleep or staying asleep due to intense thoughts and feelings	Chronic fatigue, decreased concentration, irritability

Nutrition and digestion	Increased sensitivity to certain foods	Intense physical reactions to certain foods or eating habits	Digestive problems, difficulty maintaining a balanced diet

Self management

Setting boundaries	Difficulty saying no and setting personal boundaries	Constantly wanting to help others even at the expense of one's own well-being	Exhaustion, resentment, unbalanced relationships
Self-care and recovery	Need for time and specific techniques to recharge your batteries	Need for regular practices to maintain emotional and physical balance	Neglect of self -care , emotional and physical exhaustion

Chapter 4

Managing emotions

Emotions are an integral part of daily life and understanding them is crucial. We all go through situations where we experience strong, hard-to-control emotions, but for some people, dealing with fluctuating emotions is a daily occurrence. These varying emotions can lead to impulsive behavior or impulsively spoken words that later lead to remorse. Such actions may have adverse effects on relationships or damage reputation.

Emotions have a significant influence on our daily activities by guiding our thoughts and actions and eventually our decisions. Although it may be easy to think that rationality and logic should always be at the forefront, engaging in emotional reasoning can result in wiser choices. Recognizing the impact of emotions marks the first step toward appreciating how we can harness them to our advantage. In your mind, there is one corner that remains for them: that of clandestinity.

Joy, fear, anger, sadness: emotions that run through all aspects of life. However, it is not always easy to adopt. For some, emotions can be a whirlwind that overwhelms rationality and leads to uncomfortable situations. While for others you have to bury them deep within yourself. Controlling emotions is often seen as an innate ability, but in reality, it is a skill that must be acquired.

Emotional self-regulation is what defines good emotional management: the ability to calm down, whatever the situation. This does not mean suppressing emotions; rather, it allows your emotions to guide you as intended, helping you make sense of the world around you and adapt accordingly. Additionally, emotions can serve us well if we deliberately acknowledge them and take responsibility for them while allowing them to flow freely. In order to meet these 3 challenges, we present to you 3 simple and very effective strategies that will help you manage your emotions and generally improve your emotional intelligence.

Mindfulness techniques for emotion regulation.

Mindfulness as an exercise can positively affect emotion regulation. It works by developing self-awareness, controlling emotions, reducing stress and anxiety; these are ways that allow us to manage our emotions more effectively. Mindfulness should not be practiced only during meditation or yoga, but it should be part of your daily life (short exercises and throughout the day). Although not exhaustive, the benefits of mindfulness set it apart from other options available when seeking to improve emotional regulation and are therefore worth considering and adopting.

Mindfulness is a good technique for being able to regulate your emotions. When you notice yourself feeling strong emotions, take a moment to pause and practice mindfulness. You can focus on your breathing, your body sensations, or your thoughts can help you regulate your emotions.

Ways to manage stress and anxiety. Of all these options, these solutions are beneficial for improving emotional regulation, but mindfulness has the added benefit of improving self-awareness and empathy toward oneself and others. In fact, it can be effortlessly integrated into daily life without the need for special equipment or training.

It is a set of techniques and treatments that help a person manage their stress levels. These methods can be used to ease periodic episodes of stress or treat a persistent stress disorder.

The little beast called stress: it has the capacity to sneak into our lives and create emotional turmoil. Fortunately, there are many effective methods and approaches that can help you cope with this daily stress: whether it be work or personal tasks, societal expectations, or even overwhelming cognitive load.

Every day at work, stress can feel like a terrible curse. However, efforts to manage emotions lead to self-confidence and decreased anxiety levels. Emotion and stress are closely linked . When faced with stress, we often experience feelings of anxiety, fear or even anger. The goal of managing emotions is to learn to tame these emotions and control them so as not to react aggressively.

Self-care and emotional state.
It is important to remember that the development of emotional health should be left to the discretion of each individual, should take time and require patience. Be gentle with yourself and engage in activities that promote positive emotional well-being.

Thus, it can be concluded that nurturing your emotional and mental well-being is an essential aspect of taking care of yourself holistically. There are many self-care tactics aimed at improving your emotional and mental health; it's about embracing mindfulness, interacting with the people around you, exercising regularly, and getting enough sleep. Seek professional help if necessary; learn self -compassion and limit the time you spend on screens. By valuing self-care and making strides to improve your emotional and psychological health, you have a chance to improve the quality of your life and welcome more happiness and contentment in return.

Establish a routine that involves relaxation or self-care activities to promote emotional well-being. A consistent schedule that includes activities like reading, taking a bath, listening to calming music, or practicing mindfulness within a set time limit will ensure a daily dose of relaxation and self-care. Having a predictable routine helps children feel secure and gives them time to relax and participate in activities that support their emotional health.

Seek support from others.

Be there for him emotionally, listen to his pain, help him with the appropriate authorities when needed, teach him to be assertive, build his self-esteem to high levels, show him how to seek supportive friendships.

Cultivating supportive relationships is the fourth point. It involves surrounding ourselves with people who uplift and support us, which is essential to our healing process. We should seek out friends, family, or support groups who appreciate what we are going through and validate our experiences. These relationships provide us with a safe place to talk about our thoughts and feelings; this helps create a sense of belonging and acceptance. When we cultivate supportive relationships, we build a network of people who can inspire and encourage our development without any outside input.

Solicit unprompted feedback: Make a habit of asking people you trust for their opinions on your actions and thoughts, which will help you identify places you need to change and strengthen your self-awareness with feedback. alternative perspectives of others.

Children can learn to calm their minds by engaging in relaxation and controlled breathing techniques, thereby promoting their focus on the present moment. The practice helps them eliminate external and internal distractions; this allows them to complete their tasks and activities more efficiently with increased concentration.

Learn to breathe properly: inhale deeply for a count of four, hold your breath for four, exhale for four seconds, hold your lungs empty for four seconds. This helps calm a child effectively and quickly. Let him focus on his breathing rhythm, trying to synchronize the numbers with the counts silently throughout each round. By triggering the parasympathetic nervous system through controlled deep breathing, children can feel more relaxed and have a greater sense of control over their emotions without having to use words or actions.

Category	Strategy	Description	Concrete examples

Relaxation techniques	Mindfulness meditation	Practice mindfulness to stay grounded in the present moment	Daily guided meditation, meditation apps
	Deep breathing	Use breathing techniques to calm the nervous system	Breathing 4-7-8, diaphragmatic breathing
	Progressive muscle relaxation	Gradually relax each muscle group to reduce tension	Progressive muscle relaxation exercise before sleeping
Management of thoughts	Cognitive restructuring	Identify and change negative or irrational thoughts	Keep a thought journal, work with a therapist to replace negative thoughts with positive ones
	Journaling	Write down your thoughts and emotions to clarify and understand them	Keep a daily journal, use journaling prompts to explore your emotions
	Self-compassion	Practice self - compassion to treat yourself with the same kindness you extend to others	Use positive affirmations, practice self - compassion during stressful times
Emotional expression	Art therapy	Use artistic means to express and explore your emotions	Painting, drawing, creative writing
	Movement therapy	Using movement and	Expressive dance, emotional yoga

		dance to express emotions	
	Assertive communication	Learn to express your emotions clearly and respectfully	Use "I" messages, practice active listening
Social support	Support groups	Participate in support groups to share experiences and get support	Online or in-person support groups for hypersensitive people
	Individual therapy	Working with a therapist to explore and manage your emotions	Cognitive - behavioral therapy (CBT), psychodynamic therapy
	Positive social media	Surround yourself with understanding and caring people	Maintain relationships with friends and loved ones who provide emotional support
Self-care	Hobbies	Integrate calming activities into the daily routine	Take a hot bath, read a book, listen to relaxing music
	Regular personal care	Taking care of your body to promote emotional well-being	Skin care routine, regular exercise
	Time for yourself	Plan moments of solitude to recharge your batteries	Take time for yourself every day, practice hobbies that bring joy

Advanced techniques	Movement) Therapy Desensitization and Reprocessing)	Use specific techniques to process traumatic emotions and memories	Working with an EMDR Therapist to Treat Trauma
	Biofeedback	Using biofeedback devices to learn to control physiological responses to stress	Participate in biofeedback sessions to learn how to regulate your heart rate and breathing
	Hypnotherapy	Using hypnosis to access and process underlying emotions	Working with a hypnotherapist to explore repressed emotions

Chapter 5

Development of Practical Skills

Ways to Improve Focus and Attention During Exercise

It is possible for us to build our concentration. To achieve this, we need to identify the time it takes for our brain to reach its maximum concentration level and gradually increase it. It doesn't matter how small the increment is, even if it's just five minutes more than the previous duration, for example 20 becoming 25 then 30 and so on until you can comfortably maintain your concentration for 40 to 45 minutes (already an impressive feat)! Surprisingly, after such an exercise, we find ourselves having doubled what we could call our concentrated capital without much effort; furthermore, this can be further improved given that the average time spent by individuals varies from twenty-five minutes to one hour, with the best performers going beyond two hours.

We now turn our attention to improving what we can call our concentration density or, in simple terms, our ability to focus on one thing while excluding all others. This can be significantly improved by engaging in practices like yoga, relaxation therapy and mindfulness.

Improving your concentration doesn't happen overnight. Consider the example of professional athletes such as golfers, runners and gymnasts who undergo long periods of training (often under the guidance of a coach) so that they can concentrate and perform the appropriate movements at the required time, excelling thus in their discipline.

Establishing clear boundaries in your workplace is essential. This ranges from setting physical boundaries, such as controlling light and sound in your work area, to consistently expressing your needs and expectations with your peers and superiors. It's all part of what you do. this is called relational boundary setting. It helps you deal with sensory and emotional overload, something that could easily hinder productivity if not properly managed.

Personal growth is unimaginable without self-esteem.

Observe the journey you have taken: end this step with introspection to realize everything you have learned about yourself. Consider how these revelations of your identity and values will help you lead a more enriched and harmonious life.

The desire for normalcy sets in, but what defines normality? Are these the norms we were exposed to in our youth? If being different is our individuality, then why aspire to a common "normal"? It really comes down to accepting ourselves as we are. However, it's easier said than done. Because when we express our dissatisfaction with "nothing" that resonates within us on a deep emotional level whether it is videos, movies, news, songs or even places and people triggering feelings in us varied , it becomes complex to adapt to the idea of being "normal".

Cultivate healthy lifestyle practices to improve your overall well-being.

Start your day with a few simple exercises: get your body moving. Regular exercise triggers the release of chemicals in our system that play a vital role in memory retention, improving concentration levels and sharpening mental acuity. Separate studies have also shown that physical activity can increase brain production levels of dopamine (the feel-good neurotransmitter), norepinephrine (improves mood), and serotonin (helps regulate sleep cycles). All of these play a role in attention and concentration. It is therefore not surprising that people who regularly practice sports have better cognitive performance than those who do not prioritize physical health over other aspects. Remember that when muscles move, they also relieve tension stored within them; both physically and mentally, it can help us feel lighter!

A ritual is a convergence of actions imbued with spiritual virtues, such is the essence. This prepares our mind to be efficient, to concentrate fully on our task. Everything above undoubtedly contributes to helping us achieve this state. Yet when the time comes to get down to work, we can find ourselves flirting with procrastination, delaying the start for a few extra moments, always running the incalculable risk of plunging into the abyss that is our box of receiving email.

Use these strategies to incorporate both skills into your routine.

The article may seem interesting in theory, but its practical implementation is still a challenge. Yes, having order, setting goals, and prioritizing your own tasks over others can be difficult. For example, I struggle with not responding to blog posts or resisting the urge to click on links that lead me to distractions instead of doing what I need to.

This guide delves deeper into the concept of hypersensitivity and its aspects, offering suggestions on how to better understand this particular sensitivity. The manuscript tells the history of sensitivity: it talks about the work and discoveries related to hypersensitivity, including its origins, its characteristics, and even the different pains and benefits that we get from it. Representing the daily life of very sensitive people, it focuses on their struggles, but also on revelations about what makes them unique, it draws different profiles among these individuals. There is a test included that gives you insight into your sensitivity level as well as many practical ways in which you can adjust more comfortably. Hypersensitivity problems in children and adolescents are also addressed here, with keys that could help them.

Support for skills development can help identify and highlight the unique talents of highly competent individuals, which go beyond simple intelligence to include aspects such as creative thinking or curiosity. An unconventional method for managing hypersensitivity is to practice mindfulness exercises.

There is yet another technique that proves useful: conscious breathing. Our nervous system can be put on extreme alert when we experience these episodes of hypersensitivity; however, mindful breathing can come to our rescue by helping to calm our nervous system. It achieves this by allowing us to focus on our breathing and, therefore, slow down the speed at which we breathe, allowing us to regain calm and be able to regulate our emotional reactions.

There are several ways that highly sensitive people can turn their sensitivity into a source of strength for their well-being; these include finding creative expression as well as stress management techniques. This can be achieved by fostering self-awareness, learning stress management strategies, setting boundaries, and seeking outlets for creativity.

Another way to reduce hypersensitivity triggers is to practice mindfulness that goes beyond simply sitting down to meditate. This may involve activities such as mindful walking, yoga, painting, or any other activity in which one can engage and pay full attention to what one is doing.

Category	Strategy	Description	Concrete examples
Environment			
Spatial planning	Create a dedicated and organized workspace	Keep the desk clean and tidy, use a comfortable chair	Organize the desk, eliminate distractions, add plants or calming elements
Reduction of distractions	Limit visual and auditory interruptions	Use noise-canceling headphones, put the phone on silent	Turn off notifications on phone, use distracting website blocking apps
Brightness and ergonomics	Adjust the light and ergonomics of the workspace	Use a desk lamp with natural light, adjust the height of the screen and chair	Install adequate lighting, adjust sitting posture to avoid tension
Management of time			
Time management techniques	Use methods to structure working time	Use the Pomodoro technique , schedule regular breaks	Work in 25 minute intervals with 5 minute breaks, use a timer
Prioritization of tasks	Set priorities and schedule tasks based on their importance	Using the Eisenhower Matrix, Create a Daily To-Do List	Rank tasks by urgency and importance, working on the most important tasks first
Goal Setting	Set clear, measurable goals	Use the SMART method (Specific, Measurable, Achievable, Realistic, Time-bound)	Set weekly and daily goals, track progress regularly
Concentration techniques			
Meditation and mindfulness	Practice meditation to improve concentration and mental clarity	Do daily meditation sessions, use guided meditation apps	Practice mindfulness for 10 minutes every morning, follow guided meditations

Concentration exercises	Perform specific exercises to strengthen the ability to concentrate	Play memory games, practice visual concentration exercises	Use brain training apps, practice puzzles or logic games
Conscious breathing	Use breathing techniques to calm the mind and improve concentration	Practice 4-7-8 breathing, do diaphragmatic breathing exercises	Take conscious breathing breaks between tasks, practice deep breathing
Nutrition and Hydration			
Balanced diet	Consume foods that support brain function	Eat fruits, vegetables, lean proteins, and healthy fats	Include foods rich in omega-3, avoid refined sugars and processed foods
Regular hydration	Maintain good hydration for optimal cognitive function	Drink at least 8 glasses of water per day, avoid sugary drinks	Keep a water bottle handy, set reminders to drink water
Physical activity			
Regular physical exercise	Integrate physical exercise into the daily routine	Exercise at least 30 minutes a day	Practicing walking, yoga, swimming or other physical activities regularly
Active breaks	Take breaks to move and stretch muscles	Stretch, walk during breaks	Take 5 minute breaks to walk or stretch between work sessions
Sleep and Rest			
Regular sleep routine	Establish a consistent sleep routine to promote mental recovery	Go to bed and get up at the same time every day, create a conducive sleep environment	Avoid screens before sleeping, practice calming rituals before bed
Micro-naps	Take micro-naps to recharge your energy	Take 10-20 minute naps during the day	Use guided nap apps, rest in a quiet, dark environment
Advanced techniques			

Biofeedback	Using biofeedback devices to improve concentration and emotional regulation	Participate in biofeedback sessions to learn to control physiological responses	Working with a biofeedback therapist, using biofeedback devices at home
Neurofeedback	Using neurofeedback techniques to train the brain to stay focused	Follow neurofeedback sessions with a professional	Participate in neurofeedback programs to improve cognitive functions

Chapter 6

Management Strategies for Hypersensitive Children

Hypersensitivity is a trait found in some children who are very receptive to external signals and feelings. For parents, it is essential to understand this aspect of their child's nature and help them manage it. National Hypersensitivity Day falls on January 13. We bring you five tips (supported by psychology and pedagogy professionals) that can guide you in the education of your hypersensitive child without losing any information.

Hypersensitivity is a trait that is often overlooked, but affects a large number of children. A hypersensitive child perceives stimuli in his environment more acutely than others, whether they are noises, lights, emotions or even textures. Awareness of this particularity is essential for parents, educators and professionals who work with them on a daily basis.

The increased reactivity of hypersensitive children can be observed in a variety of ways, such as overstimulation of all five senses or several senses at once. In many cases, hypersensitive children are described as feeling everything at once and being "emotional sponges." Helping these children requires establishing a safe and supportive environment that minimizes overwhelming stimuli and nurtures their emotional needs.

It is important to create a safe and comfortable place for the child to call home. Create quiet retreat spaces where the child can go when they feel overwhelmed or need time to be alone and recharge.

We will delve into all the intricacies of this unique sensitivity, from identifying signals to creating an enabling environment. Get ready to discover pragmatic advice and effective tactics that can help your highly sensitive child survive and thrive in a sometimes overwhelming world.

Sensory: Make sure the environment is as sensorially pleasant as possible. Avoid bright lights, loud noises and uncomfortable textures: opt for soft lighting, calming sounds and soft, comfortable materials. It can feel overwhelming at times.

Exercises to Help Young Children Control Their Feelings and Emotions

Help the child easily identify his feelings and call them by name. Teach him to recognize how he feels and deal with the situation in a healthy way. Motivate him to express his emotions using words instead of acting impulsively.

One strategy is to do exercises that help individuals identify their sensations and be able to predict when they will reach their emotional limit. Another strategy is to draw immediately after completing a task; the act of drawing can help calm you down by

MANAGING HYPERSENSITIVITY

focusing on the pencil strokes and colors. There are also times when he can leave the class and go to kindergarten to read a story, which allows him to regain control...

Help your child identify emotional stimuli and predict tension-producing scenarios. By helping him understand the indicators of anxiety or irritability, he can act preventively in the face of such situations.

Introduce positive encouragement and incentives.

Positive reinforcement systems have long been used by many people, both parents and educators. In a nutshell, they were studied and experimented with by psychologist Pavlov who first tested them on dogs. We introduced operant conditioning which aims to reinforce the dog's positive behavior with a reward; this technique is behavioral in the sense that it directly affects children's behavior. Since then, many have adopted such systems to reinforce existing behaviors or encourage desired behaviors in children. Opinions on these systems vary widely among individuals: some strongly argue for the effectiveness of reinforcement systems while others question its impact. Personally, I am convinced of the positive effects of these systems on children, let me explain why! But on the other hand, I also recognize that after several observations, setting up a positive reinforcement system can sometimes prove to be complex and above all to be sustained over time until a positive result is obtained in the medium or even long term. .

Another important point is to be able to see and recognize your successes, no matter how small. Let him know you appreciate what he's accomplished, no matter how big or small. This will help build his confidence and make him realize his potential to meet challenges.

Positive reinforcement plays a vital role in managing impulsivity in children. Openly acknowledge their successes with phrases like, "Good job for asking my permission before using my stuff" or "I'm proud of you for staying calm and expressing your anger gently." Acknowledging the child's efforts to control impulses can be effective, such as saying, "Thank you for waiting until instructions were completed before getting up."

Teach the child stress management strategies like deep breathing, meditation or yoga, or any other activity that promotes relaxation. Additionally, motivate him to adopt these practices consistently to strengthen his resistance to stress and sensory stimuli.

Controlling stress and anxiety is a basic requirement for any highly sensitive child. Introduce relaxation and stress control techniques. Deep breathing, meditation or yoga can be suggestions to their system when implemented to help them calm their nerves and be able to easily handle situations where they may feel stressed.

Practicality is what matters most. But it should be noted that it is also important to trigger biological and psychological responses carefully and to a reasonable extent, because not all stress reactions pose health risks. The problem arises when we are constantly under pressure without allowing ourselves the opportunity to have a natural rhythm. This can be problematic if there is no balance between the stress and relaxation phases;

however, certain signs manifested in adults (and occasionally in children) should not be ignored.

Activities adapted for hypersensitive children

Support your highly sensitive child's social development by helping him connect with friends who share his interests and engaging in activities he finds enjoyable. Open discussions with people in your environment (such as teachers or educators) to make them aware of the child's sensitivity. Also talk about preventative measures that can be adopted to ensure a supportive framework.

It may be helpful for hypersensitive children to attend workshops for hypersensitive children. These places can provide them with the tools they need to learn to better manage their sensitivity and allow them to meet other children like them who share similar traits, making them feel less alone.

Stress and frustration management skills play an important role in hypersensitive children. Practices such as meditation, coloring or breathing exercises help them keep their emotions in check and prevent overreactions.

Category	Strategy	Description	Concrete examples
Education			
Educational adaptations	Provide accommodations to support learning	Use visual supports, offer additional time for tests	Use diagrams, images, and allow more time for exams

Individualized teaching	Adapt teaching to the specific needs of the child	Offer individual tutoring sessions, adapt teaching methods	Schedule after-school tutoring sessions, use multi-sensory teaching methods
Communication with teachers	Ensure good communication between parents and teachers	Discuss the child's needs, share effective strategies	Regular meetings with teachers to monitor progress and adjust strategies

Home environment

Setting up a quiet space	Create a relaxation space at home	Arrange a bedroom or quiet corner with calming elements	Use soft colors, add comfortable cushions and blankets
Establishing Routines	Create structured routines to provide a sense of security	Establish regular schedules for meals, sleep and homework	Set up a daily schedule, use a routine chart
Limitation of sensory stimuli	Reduce disruptive sensory stimuli	Minimize loud noises, adjust brightness, avoid unpleasant textures	Use blackout curtains, earplugs, soft fabrics

Managing emotions

Relaxation techniques	Teaching relaxation methods to manage emotions	Practice deep breathing, meditation suitable for children	Use meditation apps for kids, do breathing exercises together
Creative expression	Encourage the expression of	Using art, music or writing to	Offer drawing, painting, music

	emotions through creative activities	express your feelings	or creative writing sessions
Validation of emotions	Recognize and validate the child's emotions	Actively listen, name emotions, offer emotional support	Saying "I understand you feel sad," offering hugs and comforting words
Social support			
Parent support groups	Participate in support groups to share experiences and advice	Chat with other parents of hypersensitive children	Join support groups online or in person
Strengthening family relationships	Encourage positive family activities	Spend quality time with family, practice activities together	Plan family outings, game nights or meals together
Positive social interactions	Encourage interactions with understanding and caring friends	Organize games with friends, participate in suitable group activities	Invite friends home, enroll the child in clubs or activities that interest them
health and wellbeing			
Balanced diet	Ensuring a healthy diet to support overall well-being	Offer nutrient-rich meals, avoid sugary and processed foods	Prepare homemade meals, include fruits, vegetables, proteins and whole grains
Regular physical activity	Integrate physical exercise into the daily routine	Encourage participation in	Enroll the child in dance or swimming

		active sports or games	classes, or organize family walks
Quality sleep	Ensuring good sleep to promote recovery	Establish a regular bedtime routine, create an environment conducive to sleep	Establish a calming bedtime ritual, use a soft night light, limit screens before bed

Advanced techniques

Behavioral therapy	Work with a therapist to learn emotion management techniques	Using approaches like cognitive behavioral therapy (CBT)	Consult a specialized therapist, follow a behavioral therapy program
Stress management training	Teach specific techniques for managing stress and anxiety	Use tools like stress management cards, role plays	Practice role plays to manage stressful situations, use books and adapted resources
Biofeedback	Using biofeedback devices to help the child regulate their physiological responses	Participate in biofeedback sessions to learn how to control stress responses	Work with a biofeedback professional, use child-friendly biofeedback devices

Chapter 7

Management Strategies for Hypersensitive Adults

Hypersensitivity in adults can be a fairly complex phenomenon to understand.

When we work to recognize hypersensitive adults, we delve into a detailed portrait of individuals with deep sensitivity. These particularities manifest in the physical, emotional or social domains and are influenced by the information contained in their environment. The percentage of people falling into the category of hypersensitive people amounts to 15-20%.

Perception of sensory stimuli: Hypersensitive adults have overdeveloped sensory abilities, which is why they notice stimuli in more detail and with more intensity. Sometimes this overwhelming experience can be difficult to deal with, because the five senses are very receptive to specific things like loud noises, bright lights, or strong smells (and others that usually go unnoticed by many people). Yet what you may perceive as uncomfortable due to high sensitivity can lead to confusion and stress, triggering extreme defense mechanisms such as "flight or fight." Isolation becomes the most appropriate response to these sensory attacks: it allows you to restore balance within yourself. Techniques such as meditation, breathing exercises or emotional control can be used during this time to aid recovery without any outside interference.

Increased emotional alertness: Hypersensitive adults do indeed have an increased emotional sense. The result is an experience of deeper emotions and an ease in being immersed in them, due to a rich and diverse emotional spectrum, characteristic of hyperemotivity (which is also found in high-potential individuals). Unfortunately, not everyone enjoys this emotional abundance; this can lead to deep anxiety and feelings of isolation. At such times, it is beneficial to seek companionship with other hypersensitive people who can relate to your experiences.

Foster a favorable work environment.

Promote a positive, inclusive work atmosphere that values diversity and individual abilities. It is essential to create a workspace where achievement, cooperation and a sense of respect and support are encouraged and nurtured as an integral part of the culture. Recognize the value that highly sensitive employees bring to the organization by showcasing their distinctive skills and perspectives, contributing in ways that others may not possess.

Establishing a positive work atmosphere is one of the essential tasks that effective leaders understand to be able to maintain a healthy work-life balance. Leadership style can directly affect employee well-being and productivity, but different approaches to leadership are possible. For example, transformational leadership inspires and motivates employees toward a shared vision, strengthening engagement and performance. On the other hand, servant leadership prioritizes meeting employee needs, which helps achieve a healthier work-life balance while ensuring efficiency. Whichever way it is chosen, make sure that the approach used allows each employee to feel valued and supported: choose a leadership style carefully.

The Harvard Business Review states that good work environments improve employee satisfaction and productivity, making for a productive and satisfied workforce. Consider spaces that foster creativity through collaboration, where ideas can flow easily among team members informally. Modern break rooms, relaxation zones, green spaces: companies are starting to introduce such elements into their workspace in order to show that they care about providing a low-stress, high-involvement environment.

Think about communication strategies to apply when dealing with hypersensitive staff. Use precise language, short and concise words; do not shout or speak violently, but rather provide positive criticism with care and sensitivity. Changing the way you communicate can lead to building an appreciative relationship and promoting a spirit of cooperation in this particular situation.

An essential action to promote healthy relationships involves regularly organizing team meetings where both strategic and operational information is shared. It is possible to maintain communication with employees without overloading calendars by holding brief weekly meetings; These meetings can be a great forum for communicating positive events to all team members. The birth of a child or a letter of congratulations received by a member of the team are events which, in agreement with the employees concerned, could be shared among other things to strengthen mutual understanding within the group. Such meetings will guarantee everyone's involvement in these details: professional and personal.

First mention goes to active listening, an essential part of effective communication that helps both parties feel recognized and understood. Nonviolent communication commonly addressed in workshops equipped with specialized tools to express personal needs without hostility is the second mention. The third is empathy, fundamental to recognizing the emotions and divergent points of view of others. When conflict prevention involves promoting respectful and empathetic communication, it deters conflicts from escalating. Showing sensitivity on these points can improve your conflict management skills and cultivate a more peaceful coexistence.

Stress management techniques must be adopted and applied.

There are many practical techniques and tools to combat stress on a daily basis. On the one hand, breathing exercises, such as meditation, are effective in helping you return to a calm and peaceful state of mind. You only need 5 minutes each day; you just need to clarify your thoughts and emotions.

Strategy must be at the top of the list: these managers must adopt stress management techniques. This includes, but is not limited to, meditating, mindfulness, or taking planned breaks during the day; this helps curb this overstimulation and maintain a healthy mental state.

In the professional field, stress management is synonymous with the ability to control oneself in the face of high-pressure scenarios and tides of tension. But it is also about knowing how to let go, adopting an air of tranquility even in the midst of irritating or unexpected situations. These behavioral skills can be acquired through personal development work. Dive into managing your emotions so that you don't lash out aggressively, but rather maintain your composure in stressful circumstances. Stress management therefore acts as a pivot: converting stress into positive energy which can find application in the professional sphere and reverberate in the private and family domains.

Promote self-care and find work-life balance. A good work-life balance can help you build resilience and minimize stress in all areas of your life. Remember the recommendations listed below; choose the ones that best suit your situation. Experiment with an idea: It's like testing a single suggestion, so you'll come back for more thoughts.

Maintaining balance is the key to a healthy personal and professional life. Here are some original suggestions to help you find your balance on an individual level. Be sure to pass them on to your boss; they can spark an idea that could revolutionize work-life balance for all staff members.

Don't hesitate to ask for help and accept the support that is offered to you. Simply opening up to another person about your struggles can alleviate a significant portion of your stress. You are not alone on this journey: be open to seeking, receiving, and accepting support.

Practical exercises for hypersensitive adults

Let me share a few more techniques that work wonders. In times of intense anxiety, I have a solitary session, standing in front of a mirror, where I talk to myself, offering words of comfort and empowerment. Another practice is to dedicate a few moments at night, in bed, to communicating with my subconscious, my body and my "superego" (including education and principles) to work in unison. This helps me to retrospectively analyze my responses with more composure and preemptively manage or control them in future instances.

The resource aims to offer a variety of exercises including expression games, listening games, attention and concentration games, relaxation activities and visualization activities. These exercises can be carried out in different contexts: inside or outside the classroom or even the school. The timing of these exercises could be at the start of the day to start positively, after a high-intensity motor activity, following moments of tension or emotion. The planned exercises aim to help the learner: improve their concentration; stir up his vigor; relax without strength; untie physical knots effortlessly; unveil hidden power and determination; refine the auditory senses; sharpen visual perception skills; refine effective communication strategies; stimulate cognitive faculties with stimulating tasks; giving vent to one's feelings through emotional expression; bring the body to greater flexibility, also nourishing it; nourish a feeling of well-being.

Experiment with touch: close your eyes and run your palm over the bark of a tree. Breathe deeply while holding this posture for at least ninety seconds. The contact of raw wood with your palm has a tranquillizing effect on the activity of your prefrontal cortex; it initiates parasympathetic nervous action, leading to physiological relaxation. In addition, the bark is bactericidal, meaning it kills bacteria. So when you touch the tree, you also help protect it. Close your eyes and feel the texture under your palm; take a deep breath and let nature do its work as you drift off into tranquility.

Category	Strategy	Description	Concrete examples
Managing emotions			
Mindfulness meditation	Practice mindfulness to stay grounded in the present moment	Do daily meditation sessions, use guided meditation apps	Practice mindfulness for 10 minutes every morning, follow guided meditations
Breathing techniques	Use breathing techniques to calm the nervous system	Practice 4-7-8 breathing, do diaphragmatic breathing exercises	Take conscious breathing breaks between tasks, practice deep breathing
Journaling	Write down your thoughts and emotions to clarify and understand them	Keep a daily journal, use journaling prompts to explore your emotions	Write every evening about the events of the day and your feelings
Environment			
Spatial planning	Create a calm and organized work or living space	Keep the desk clean and tidy, use a comfortable chair	Organize the desk, eliminate distractions, add plants or calming elements
Reduction of sensory stimuli	Minimize loud noises, adjust brightness, avoid unpleasant textures	Use noise-canceling headphones, put the phone on silent	Turn off notifications on phone, use distracting website blocking apps

Establishing Routines	Create structured routines to provide a sense of security	Establish regular schedules for meals, sleep and work	Set up a daily schedule, use a routine chart
Social relations			
Assertive communication	Learn to express your emotions clearly and respectfully	Use "I" messages, practice active listening	Say "I feel…" instead of "You make me feel…", listen attentively without interrupting
Limiting social interactions	Retreating from social interactions to recharge	Schedule alone time after intense social events	Carve out some alone time after a meeting or party
Strengthening positive relationships	Surround yourself with understanding and caring people	Maintain relationships with friends and loved ones who provide emotional support	Spend time with close friends, avoid toxic people
Time and Stress Management			
Time management techniques	Use methods to structure working time	Use the Pomodoro technique , schedule regular breaks	Work in 25 minute intervals with 5 minute breaks, use a timer
Prioritization of tasks	Set priorities and schedule tasks based on their importance	Using the Eisenhower Matrix, Create a Daily To-Do List	Rank tasks by urgency and importance, working on the most important tasks first

Self-compassion	Practice self - compassion to treat yourself with the same kindness you extend to others	Use positive affirmations, practice self - compassion during stressful times	Tell yourself "I'm doing my best" when you make mistakes or fail, take time for yourself

Health and wellbeing

Balanced diet	Consume foods that support brain function and emotional stability	Eat fruits, vegetables, lean proteins, and healthy fats	Include foods rich in omega-3, avoid refined sugars and processed foods
Regular physical activity	Integrate physical exercise into the daily routine	Exercise at least 30 minutes a day	Practicing walking, yoga, swimming or other physical activities regularly
Quality sleep	Ensuring good sleep to promote mental recovery	Establish a regular bedtime routine, create an environment conducive to sleep	Establish a calming bedtime ritual, use a soft night light, limit screens before bed

Advanced Techniques

Behavioral therapy	Work with a therapist to learn emotion management techniques	Using approaches like cognitive behavioral therapy (CBT)	Consult a specialized therapist, follow a behavioral therapy program
Stress management training	Use tools and exercises to learn to manage stress	Use stress management apps, practice relaxation exercises	Participate in stress management workshops, use relaxation

			techniques such as visualization
Biofeedback	Using biofeedback devices to help regulate one's physiological responses	Participate in biofeedback sessions to learn how to control stress responses	Working with a biofeedback professional, using biofeedback devices at home

Chapter 8

Therapeutic and Medical Approaches

Therapies such as behavioral and cognitive approaches are interventions against mental distress that follow a methodology directly born from the experimental method applied to an individual case. These approaches are now widely recognized, both by the general public and by health professionals, and are recommended for various psychological disorders. For example, a basic postulate of cognitive behavioral therapy (CBT) views maladaptive behavior (such as a phobia) as drawn from past experiences in similar situations; this behavior then appears to be perpetuated by environmental contingencies.

He adopts an integrative therapeutic approach: this implies that he will select the most suitable methods and techniques. Whether it is cognitive -behavioral therapy (CBT) to address your thought patterns, a humanistic approach aimed at improving your personal growth or psychodynamics diving into the roots of your difficulties, even therapy oriented towards solutions seeking to identify practical solutions will focus on you. No matter what these approaches discover about you, they will improve it.

CBT, or cognitive behavioral therapy, explores the complex workings of an individual's thought patterns and actions. It enlightens the patient on why he adopts these specific behaviors in his daily life. Unlike other forms of therapy, the cognitive approach looks for current triggers for problematic behaviors, with the ultimate goal of fostering lasting change. The therapist therefore orients himself towards healing the disorders not by superficial means, but by transforming the thoughts, behaviors and emotions of the patient; an approach where success is measured by this fundamental criterion.

In the treatment of hypersensitivity, there are two options: magnetic stimulation therapy or psychotherapy, which the doctor recommends based on the assessment of the patient's condition. It is advisable to seek advice from a certified clinical psychologist who can approve this choice and suggest another effective solution to treat other diseases associated with hypersensitivity if they appear.

Various medical methodologies can be used to treat side effects resulting from hypersensitivity. The choice of treatment depends on the diagnosis and specific symptoms related to hypersensitivity.

Drug treatment proves its effectiveness in cases of hypersensitivity where symptoms manifest strongly, preventing the individual from functioning normally or causing significant disruption in daily life. However, the hypersensitive person may experience increased anxiety at the mere thought of ingesting the medication, further exacerbating symptoms of anxiety and depression. It is crucial that this person first adjusts the dosage that suits their body dynamics and timing, ensuring gradual cessation if necessary. Additionally, for those who unfortunately do not respond due to inherent hypersensitivity to medications, magnetic stimulation therapy (which is a non-drug-based alternative) is another viable approach.

Psychodynamic and humanistic approaches focus on the positive aspects of an individual's psyche. They emphasize a person's well-being rather than focusing solely on their problems or shortcomings. Through genuine caring and empathy, these approaches facilitate confidential, non-judgmental interactions in every session.

Since each individual is intrinsically complex and distinct, methodologies must be flexible and multiple in order to conform to each individual and their specific odyssey through life. There is no panacea, but diverse strategies that can reveal each person's innate personal reservoirs, on which we can count for metamorphosis, innovation, change or even leisure: a life cut in our image.

GESTALT therapy is part of the humanist and existential waves: it seeks the personal, psychosocial and organizational metamorphosis of the individual. It explores the dynamic between you as a person and your environment; The essence of this therapy is to help you understand how you construct meaning in your present moment of life, by working on your physical entity, your cognitive processes and your affective experiences. By allowing the patient to follow their own path, this approach helps them make meaningful life choices.

Strategies such as adopting lifestyle changes and alternative therapies may be considered to combat hypersensitivity. However, if the difficulties in daily life due to this disease as well as its distressing symptoms persist and do not subside even after taking self-help measures, including voluntary relaxation, it is advisable to go to a psychosomatic medicine or psychiatry department for a detailed medical evaluation. Although the first diagnostic session requires several examinations before determining treatment methods, it also helps identify other possible underlying conditions contributing to your hypersensitivity.

Simply put: managing emotional hypersensitivity can be a real challenge, but if you can tailor a treatment plan that works for you and take control of your lifestyle, it is possible to alleviate these symptoms. Sophrology and the stimulation of acupuncture points go hand in hand, they support you both physically and emotionally, helping to reduce stress levels, balance your emotions and make you more peaceful in everyday situations. It is a learning process that takes time and effort; however, with the support of your family, your friends or even professionals, these different methods will teach you to better manage your emotions in the long term.

To prevent hypersensitivity reactions, here are some tactics.

Creating a sense of security for people struggling with low confidence and hypersensitivity can be an effective way to manage their condition. This allows them to lead a comfortable and stress-free life promoting peace of mind.

A large number of (hyper)sensitive individuals are therefore completely engulfed and unable to organize the mental processes created by these stimulations; they lose their sense of direction. Now the first response will be to stop logically analyzing the situation and let your emotions take control.

Understanding hypersensitivity is an art. But when you understand it well, you will be able to accept it. Hypersensitivity does not exist in isolation. It's a reaction, a response. Knowing this can help us unlock our potential while accepting its reality. We have many sources to guide us on this journey: documentary materials, personal testimonies, and even conversations with other hypersensitive people who can share their experiences and wisdom.

Category	Approach	Description	Concrete examples
Behavioral Therapy			
Cognitive Behavioral Therapy (CBT)	Helps change negative thought patterns and develop strategies for managing emotions and behaviors	Work with a CBT therapist to identify and change dysfunctional thoughts and behaviors	
Dialectical Behavior Therapy (DBT)	Combines behavioral therapy and mindfulness techniques to manage intense emotions	Use emotional regulation, distress tolerance and mindfulness techniques	
Talk Therapy			
Psychodynamic Therapy	Explores past emotions and experiences to understand current emotional patterns	Work with a therapist to explore internal conflicts and past experiences	
Humanist Therapy	Emphasizes personal growth and self-acceptance	Using person-centered approaches to promote self-expression and acceptance	
Creative Therapy			
Art Therapy	Uses art to express and process emotions	Participate in painting, drawing or sculpture sessions led by an art therapist	
Music therapy	Use music to explore and manage emotions	Using music, singing or playing instruments to express feelings	
Movement Therapy			
Dance Therapy	Uses movement and dance to express and process emotions	Participate in dance therapy sessions to use the body as a means of emotional expression	

Therapeutic Yoga	Combines yoga postures with breathing and meditation techniques to promote emotional regulation	Practice yoga with an instructor trained in therapeutic yoga

Somatic Therapy

EMDR Therapy (Eye Movement Desensitization and Reprocessing)	Treats trauma and intense emotions using guided eye movements	Working with an EMDR therapist to process traumatic memories or intense emotions
Somatic Experiencing	Uses bodily sensations to address trauma and emotional tension	Participate in somatic therapy sessions to explore bodily sensations and release tension

Relaxation Techniques

Biofeedback	Uses devices to learn to control physiological responses to stress	Participate in biofeedback sessions to learn how to regulate breathing, heart rate and blood pressure
Mindfulness Meditation	Use mindfulness to stay grounded in the present moment and reduce stress	Practice mindfulness meditation daily, use guided meditation apps

Medical Approaches

Anxiolytic Drugs	Medications to reduce anxiety and promote relaxation	Using doctor-prescribed anti-anxiety medications to manage anxiety symptoms
Antidepressants	Medications to treat depression and anxiety disorders	Using prescribed antidepressants to balance neurotransmitter levels in the brain

Nutritional Therapy

Consultation with a Nutritionist	Adapt diet to promote emotional and physical well-being	Work with a nutritionist to develop a balanced, nutrient-rich eating plan
Food Supplements	Using Supplements to Support Mental and Emotional Health	Take omega-3, magnesium, or other supplements recommended by a healthcare professional
Social Support		
Support Groups	Participate in support groups to share experiences and advice	Join online or in-person support groups for hypersensitive people
Group Therapy	Participate in group therapy sessions to explore emotions and behaviors with other people	Work with a group therapist to share experiences and coping strategies

Chapter 9

Create a Favorable Environment

Dealing with hypersensitivity makes life difficult to live on a daily basis; however, it is possible to design an enabling environment that can help better address these challenges. The following tips show you how to adapt the school environment for highly sensitive people, develop an inclusive work environment for them and ensure that relationships at home remain harmonious.

Organize your personal space to reduce stress

Arranging personal space is a key element in reducing stress in hypersensitive people. Here are some strategies:

Color Choices: Soft hues that whisper tranquility when splashed on walls are known to create an air of peace. The soft neutrality of pastels is often favored in such cases.

Let the light be, but not too bright: ban harsh fluorescent lights from your space and enjoy the glow of natural light as much as possible. Opt for dimmable alternatives for versatility and ambiance.

Order breeds serenity; minimalism breeds focus: chaos breeds anxiety, just as disorder breeds distraction. Keep visual noise at bay by ruling over your environment with a minimalist scepter: every object must deserve its place. After all, a lesson in organization is a lesson in mindfulness.

Transform into a reading nook: One way to create quiet resting areas is to transform it into a reading nook with cushions and soft blankets. This will provide a calming sanctuary.

Create an appropriate school environment for hypersensitive students. The school environment can be overly stimulating, especially for highly sensitive students.
Here are some adjustments that can be made to help these people:
Quiet Zones: Make sure you have quiet corners where students can retreat when they feel overwhelmed.

Change the physical layout of the classroom to accommodate individual preferences, such as sitting alone or without a partner, because some students learn better this way.

Use visual aids and sound cues in addition to verbal instructions so you don't make learning stressful because of those who don't understand just the words.

Teachers and students are always advised to speak freely, so that if there are any special needs, they can be met without delay.

A work environment that embraces all differences and takes into account different needs:
To build an ideal work environment in the professional context, it is essential to consider everyone's feelings and emotions that they bring to work with them. Here are some suggestions:

Schedule Flexibility: Offering flexible work hours can help highly sensitive employees manage their energy levels and stress more effectively.

Work environment: Establish quiet work areas, free from noise pollution or enclosed spaces created by partitions within an open office space.

Psychological support: Initiate psychological support mechanisms such as counseling sessions or group therapy.

Develop training and awareness: Empower staff and leaders with knowledge about hypersensitivity, establishing an environment that promotes inclusion and respect.

Suggestions for Cultivating Harmony in Personal Relationships
Fostering peace in personal relationships is essential to the well-being of highly sensitive people. Here are some ideas:

Nonviolent Communication: Embrace nonviolent communication as a tool to express your needs without hostility, while listening to others without defensiveness or criticism.

Routine and predictability: Having a consistent habitual behavior can significantly reduce the psychological impact of apprehension of the unknown or sudden changes without warning.

Quality Time: Share quality time together, while recognizing and respecting each other's need for personal space to rejuvenate their energy levels.

Understanding and support: Foster an environment based on empathy and solidarity, where each member of the family feels valued for their uniqueness and their concerns heard.

Creating a supportive environment for highly sensitive people is an achievable outcome if these tactics are put in place, they aim to help these people manage their daily lives and reduce their stress, ultimately leading to their overall well-being.

Category	Strategy	Description	Concrete examples
Living space			
Setting up a quiet space	Create quiet areas to recharge your batteries	Use calming colors, comfortable furniture and natural elements	Set up a reading corner with cushions, use indoor plants to bring serenity
Reduction of sensory stimuli	Minimize loud noises, adjust brightness, avoid unpleasant textures	Use blackout curtains, soft rugs, white noise diffusers	Install curtains to control light, use earplugs or noise-canceling headphones
Organization and storage	Keep the living space clean and orderly	Use storage systems to avoid clutter and visual stress	Use storage baskets, shelves and boxes to organize items
Workspace			
Creating an ergonomic workspace	Create a comfortable and functional workspace	Use an ergonomic chair, adjust the height of the screen and chair	Install a height-adjustable desk, use a laptop stand
Limiting distractions	Reduce visual and auditory interruptions	Use screens or panels to separate the workspace, turn off notifications	Install screens to create visual separation, use website blocking applications
Routine and Habits			
Establishing Regular Routines	Create daily routines to provide structure	Establish regular schedules for	Use a schedule, follow a morning and night routine

	and a sense of security	meals, sleep, and daily activities	
Break planning	Take regular breaks to rest and recharge	Plan moments of relaxation and recovery throughout the day	Take a 5-minute break every hour, stretch or walk outside
Technologies and Tools			
Use of relaxation technologies	Use apps and tools to promote relaxation and reduce stress	Use meditation apps, essential oil diffusers, dim lights	Use a guided meditation app, diffuse relaxing essential oils
Control of screens and blue light	Reduce exposure to blue light from screens to improve sleep and reduce eye strain	Use blue light filters, limit screen use before sleeping	Install blue light filters on screens, use anti-blue light glasses
Physical Well-being			
Regular physical activity	Integrate physical exercise into the daily routine	Practicing gentle physical activities such as yoga, walking or swimming	Take online yoga classes, take a daily walk
Balanced diet	Consume foods that support brain function and emotional stability	Eat fruits, vegetables, lean proteins, and healthy fats	Prepare homemade meals, include foods rich in omega-3
Social Support			
Strengthening positive relationships	Surround yourself with understanding and caring people	Maintain relationships with friends and loved	Spend time with close friends, avoid toxic people

		ones who provide emotional support	
Limiting stressful social interactions	Retreat after intense social interactions to recharge	Schedule alone time after intense social events	Carve out some alone time after a meeting or party
Stress management			
Relaxation techniques	Use relaxation techniques to reduce stress and anxiety	Practice deep breathing, meditation, progressive muscle relaxation	Use meditation apps, do breathing exercises
Creative activities	Using art, music or writing to express your feelings	Participate in painting, drawing, writing or music sessions	Do painting or drawing sessions at home, write in a journal

Chapter 10

Resources and Support

Hypersensitivity can be a daunting task, but there are many resources and supports available to help people better manage this condition. An overview of support groups, other resources, specialized organizations and suggestions for finding a therapist or counselor.

Support groups and online communities

Support groups and online communities provide a safe place for individuals to tell their stories and receive support:

Forums and social media: There are many forums and groups on social media that address hypersensitivity. They provide a space where you can seek opinions, tell stories, or simply find an empathetic ear.

Meetup Groups : A few other platforms facilitate gatherings of people who identify as highly sensitive, whether in physical or virtual environments; here, individuals can connect with others and exchange notes on coping mechanisms.

Books and resources on hypersensitivity:
Many organizations are hosting webinars and virtual meetings focused on hypersensitivity, providing viewers with expert opinions as well as discussion leads.

Additional books and resources
Books and other educational resources can provide an in-depth understanding of hypersensitivity and strategies for managing it:

Articles and blogs: Many blogs and articles populate the Internet, written by experts or hypersensitive individuals, telling their personal stories interspersed with advice.

Podcasts and videos: Join discussions, listen to stories about hypersensitivity, or learn coping skills through podcasts or YouTube channels.

Organizations and associations dedicated to hypersensitivity
Many groups and associations have been created with the sole aim of showing their support for hypersensitive people and raising awareness of this pathology among the general public:

The Highly Sensitive People (HSP) Network: This particular organization has a wealth of resources, information, as well as support groups specifically designed for highly sensitive people.

Sensitive and Thriving: This is an online community that aims to help highly sensitive people thrive through workshops, resources, and coaching.

Guidelines for finding a specialized therapist or counselor

Finding a mental health professional specializing in hypersensitivity can greatly contribute to the effective management of this condition:

Web search: Use search engines to find therapists who specialize in hypersensitivity.

Recommendations can come from friends, family, or online support groups. Professional psychology associations often offer directories of certified and specialized therapists on their websites. It is advisable to meet the therapist during a first appointment and talk about your hypersensitivity. During this session, you will be able to assess whether the therapist has the necessary experience and skills that would benefit you.

Highly sensitive people can find effective ways to manage their situation and improve their quality of life by using these materials and seeking support.

30 day program

Day	Objective	Activities
1	**Initial assessment**	- Do a self-assessment of your hypersensitivity - Note the situations and main triggers of your sensitivity
2	**Create a calming space**	- Create a quiet corner at home with calming elements (plants, soft light, comforting objects)
3	**Introduction to Mindfulness**	- Practice 10 minutes of mindfulness meditation
4	**Management of time**	- Plan your week with regular breaks to rest and recover
5	**Breathing techniques**	- Learn and practice deep breathing exercises
6	**Sensory sensitivity**	- Identify sources of sensory stress (noises, lights, textures) and find solutions to alleviate them
7	**Physical activity**	- Incorporate 30 minutes of gentle exercise such as yoga or walking

8	**Emotional Journal**	- Start a journal to record your daily emotions and thoughts
9	**Balanced nutrition**	- Plan healthy and balanced meals for the week
10	**Advanced mindfulness**	- Practice 15 minutes of mindfulness meditation, focusing on your bodily sensations
11	**Limiting negative stimuli**	- Reduce the time spent on social media or watching stressful news
12	**Development of social skills**	- Learn assertive communication techniques to express your needs and limits
13	**Creating a Sleep Routine**	- Establish a regular bedtime routine with soothing activities (reading, warm bath)
14	**Reflection and self-compassion**	self-compassion and gratitude exercises
15	**Managing emotions**	- Learn techniques for managing intense emotions, such as self-soothing and grounding
16	**Creative activity**	- Spend time on a creative activity that fascinates you (drawing, music, writing)

17	Positive socialization	- Plan a meeting with supportive friends or loved ones
18	Relaxation techniques	- Learn and practice progressive muscle relaxation techniques
19	Use of art therapy	- Experiment with art therapy to express and understand your emotions
20	Limitation of commitments	- Review your social and professional commitments and learn to say no to excessive demands
21	Active listening practice	- Practice active listening in your conversations to improve your relationships and reduce misunderstandings
22	Management of sensory stress	- Use earplugs or sleep masks to reduce disruptive sensory stimuli
23	Creating a Recovery Plan	- Develop a plan for days when you feel particularly overwhelmed, including calming activities and rest time
24	Positive reinforcement	- Set up a reward system to encourage you to adopt sensitivity management habits

25	**Nature Exploration**	- Spend time outdoors, walk in nature, observe plants and animals
26	**Visualization techniques**	- Practice positive visualization exercises to reduce anxiety and stress
27	**Evaluating progress**	- Review your notes and reflections from previous days to assess your progress
28	**Adjusting strategies**	- Adjust your sensitivity management strategies based on the results of your assessment
29	**Strengthening relationships**	- Invest time in positive and enriching relationships
30	**Long-term planning**	- Establish a long-term management plan to maintain your progress and continue to improve your quality of life

QUIZ

Answer the following questions with "Yes" or "No" to assess whether you have signs of hypersensitivity. This quiz is for informational purposes and does not replace a professional diagnosis.

Emotional sensitivity

Do you often feel intense emotions, whether joy, sadness, or anger?

Do you tend to cry easily, even for reasons that others might consider minor?

Are you deeply touched by works of art, music, or nature?

Increased empathy

Do you often feel other people's emotions as if they were your own?

Do you find it difficult to watch violent or emotionally charged scenes on television or in movies?

Do you have trouble saying no to others for fear of hurting or disappointing them?

Sensory sensitivity

Are you easily disturbed by loud noises, bright lights, or unpleasant textures?

Do you find certain environments (like crowds or shopping malls) particularly exhausting or stressful?

Do you have a strong reaction to physical pain or discomfort?

Deep reflection

Do you spend a lot of time thinking about the meaning of events in your life and your own feelings?

Do you have a vivid and detailed imagination, sometimes to the point of feeling overwhelmed by your thoughts?

Do you tend to anticipate the consequences of your actions in great detail?

Need for solitude and recovery

Do you often feel the need to isolate yourself to recover after being socially active ?

Do you find that spending time alone helps you recharge and feel better?

Do you sometimes avoid social interactions or group activities because they are too exhausting?

Results

If you answered "Yes" to several questions in each section, you may be hypersensitive.

If you answered "Yes" to a few questions in one or two sections, you might have hypersensitive traits without it being dominant in your life.

Conclusion

Hypersensitivity is a complex and profound characteristic that influences many aspects of daily life. Through this book, we have explored the many facets of hypersensitivity, its unique challenges, and the many ways to manage it and positively integrate it into our lives.

First, it is essential to recognize that hypersensitivity is not a weakness, but a difference. It is a way of interacting with the world that, although sometimes taxing, also brings emotional richness and depth of perception. Highly sensitive people feel emotions more intensely, pick up on the subtleties of human relationships, and are often deeply touched by art and nature.

However, this heightened sensitivity can also make social interactions, stimulating environments, and stressful situations more difficult to manage. We therefore discussed various strategies to navigate these challenges: relaxation techniques, arrangement of living and working space, development of calming routines, and use of mindfulness.

Self-compassion is another key theme in this book. Learning to treat yourself with kindness and accept your emotions without judgment is fundamental for hypersensitive people. It is crucial to create spaces where we can recharge and find comfort.

We also emphasized the importance of positive relationships. Being surrounded by understanding and caring people can make a big difference. Whether through friends, family or support groups, the social network plays a crucial role in the well-being of hypersensitive people.

Ultimately, hypersensitivity is a valuable part of your identity. By learning to understand and manage this trait, you can turn your challenges into strengths and enrich your life significantly. This book is just a starting point. Keep exploring, learning and growing.

Thank you for joining me on this journey. I hope the knowledge and tools shared here will help you fully embrace your hypersensitivity and make it a valuable asset in your life.

Take care of yourself, and remember: sensitivity is strength.

Best wishes !

What did you think of it?

Leaving your review about the book on Amazon, even if it is brief, helps us enormously.

So even if it is only a few words, I would be extremely grateful if you would leave me your feelings in a comment.

To do so, scan the QR code below or log in to your Amazon account, click on Orders, find this book, and finally, click on the Write a review button.

Thanks

I would like to express my gratitude to the people who made this book possible.

I also thank my friends who have been an important source of inspiration in relation to the problems encountered on a daily basis. Sharing our experiences has been very enriching from a personal point of view.

Thank you to the readers, hoping that this book can give you the keys to combat hypersensitivity.

Copyright